Klaus Kampmann

Power Napping

How a 10 minute daily nap can

improve your performance and health

1st Edition 2020
© Klaus Kampmann, Texts,
Illustrations, Envelope

Author: Klaus Kampmann
Berlin, Germany

ISBN: 9798649779272
Imprint: Independently published

Table of content

Introduction

Stress, overstrain and burn-out are increasingly occurring phenomena in today's society. These can sometimes lead to high blood pressure and to the weakening of the immune system. Even with 10–30 minutes of napping, the so-called power nap, these symptoms can be removed or counteracted. The secret lies in the relaxation that comes with sleep in between. After that, the body is more rested, the mood is uplifted and the general condition improves.

The generations before us have already indulged themselves in the midday sleep. Was it possible, that they laid down after eating lunch to sleep.? It is assumed that for this reason this generation was more relaxed and in a better mood than we are today.

Power Nap: Everything speaks for it — nothing against it. That's why you should take care of your daily lunch sleep.

In this book you will learn everything you need to know to prepare and implement your power naps optimally.

Chapter 1 Basic knowledge Power Nap

Recreational sleep is not an invention of modern times. In famous paintings by the old masters there is always the motif of the sleeping person during the day. The 1565 painting 'The Harvesters' by Pieter Bruegel the Elder (exhibition venue The Metropolitan Museum of Art, New York) shows farmers eating, sleeping and resting. Others, on the other hand, pursue their work on a very hot day. Sleeping in public spaces while waiting for something, for example, was still considered normal just two generations ago.

Unfortunately, in today's society it is no longer socially acceptable to power nap during working hours. Naps are generally frowned upon and few have the courage to indulge in it. It is often regarded as a sign of weakness and therefore it is avoided. One wants to be productive and look good in front of others. You workday and night and take care of your own health. Some people don't take a break at all during the day, as they think they can make better progress. But it is precisely in this thinking that lies the mistake. You can only work efficiently if the body and mind are in the sound. That's why it's so important to treat yourself and give yourself enough breaks.

At present, various organizations around the world have failed to introduce office sleep, because good will is slowed down by the collective bad conscience. You don't sleep at work, especially in front of your colleagues.

Against this background, executives have a double chance to establish power napping in operation. They benefit themselves from the short-term recovery sleep and their employees also. It can be assumed that implementation leads to a change in interaction with each other and to greater respect and appreciation of the individual. Communication among each other will benefit from this. One indication that this may be so is a study by Dr. William D. S. Killgore, Associate Professor of Psychology, Harvard Medical School. Too little sleep causes a bad mood and a destructive coexistence: There is simply a lack of emotional intelligence.

Increased performance, increased concentration and decision-making, faster processing of complex tasks, increased creativity and an increased resilience are good arguments for the use of short-term sleep.

Those who rush themselves and who suffer from constant stress need methods to get rid of its negative consequences. This is where napping comes in. As naps should last only about 20 minutes and provides optimal relaxation, it is perfect for relieving stress.

What is a Power Nap?

Many people wonder what a Power Nap really is. A power nap is essentially a short sleep which restores. If someone has nodded in for a few minutes, then bending the head down – the typical posture for a short-term sleep – is meant. The best time to keep this short nap is usually between 12:00 and 15:00. In this period, conductivity is the lowest in many people. With a Power Nap you can recharge the energy storage.

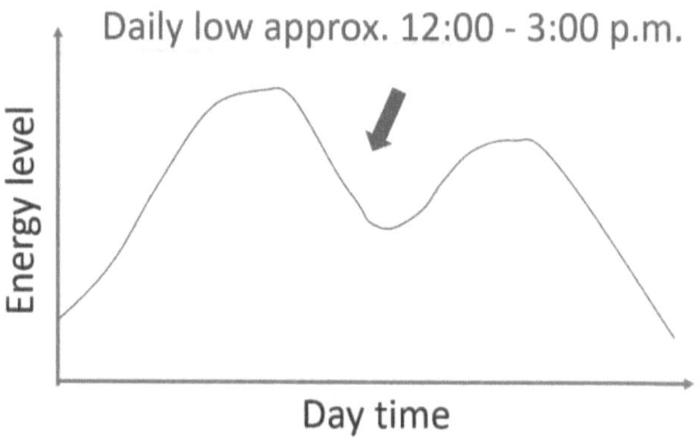

The midday low is more influenced by body rhythms than by the digestion of lunch.

The energy curve of the day looks in most people, as shown in the sketch. Typical is a decrease in performance at lunchtime. Chronobiologists have disproved the popular belief that this is related to the midday. The power curve follows the inner biorhythm: However, additional digestion increases the energy drop. Thus, the observation of previous generations is already correct, only today we know more details regarding the origin. In three-group trials, participants received at lunchtime a) nothing to eat, b) a light diet and c) heavy food. The subjects of all three groups had a lunchtime sleep on their own. The decisive difference was the duration of the nap. People who had eaten something slept 90 minutes, while fasting slept only 30 minutes. Both are basically good sleep lengths. 30 minutes is the maximum time for a nap before falling into deep sleep. 90 minutes is an entire sleep cycle with all four sleep phases. This attempt was published in the Sleep Journal in 1995 by Gary Zammit, head of the Sleep Disorder Institute in New York.

The Power Nap is defined as a short-term sleep and therefore does not last as long as the night sleep. The most common forms are 10-30 minutes. This short time is enough to stimulate and execute a variety of processes that increase performance. The ultimate time span for a Power Nap is seen in the duration of a complete sleep cycle – about 1.5 hours. The lowest limit is about five minutes.

For Power Nap there are some other common expressions: power nap, short-term sleep, nap, mini sleep, power-sleep, doze, siesta, inemuri or energy sleep.

By contrast, chilling so popular today is not a nap. It is a rest without sleeping, and thus does not have the same profound effect as a Power Nap.

What are the benefits of napping?

A short nap is not a replacement for the night's sleep, but it is astonishing the enormous positive effect of a relatively short daytime sleep on the organism the brain and the mood. If we take about 20 minutes to doze off, then nature gives us a whole range of advantages. Medical research is evidence of the health effect of power napping.

Short-term sleep decreases blood pressure and body temperature. Hormonal changes are made, which give us the right kick for the afternoon after sleep.

Decades of research at the Harvard School of Public Health have shown that regular siesta (3 x 30 minutes per week) lowers the risk of heart attack by up to 37%. The long-term study included 24,000 people in Greece. The effect is achieved, among other things, because stress hormones are vastly reduced during sleep and blood pressure and heart rhythm is able to recover.

It is worth taking a nap for health, fitness and cognitive performance.

15 arguments for short-term sleep:

1.... positive effect on health.

2.... lowers blood pressure.

3.... lowers the risk of heart disease.

4.... increases performance and responsiveness.

5.... relieves stress.

6.... reduces errors.

7.... reduces the risk of accidents.

8.... increases the ability to concentrate and learn.

9.... improves overall mood.

10.... increases the load capacity.

11.... strengthens the immune system.

12.... promotes decision-making power.

13.... increases will-power.

14.... can give you bursts of energy.

15.... may reduce the risk of Alzheimer's.

Famous people such as Leonardo Da Vinci, Napoleon Bonaparte, Johannes Brahms, Thomas Edison, Albert Einstein, Salvador Dali and many more have taken advantage of the benefits of lunch. There are demonstrably a large number of flashes of mind that have made the way from the most unconscious depths of the brain to the surface when taking a nap. It is known from Isaac Newton that the falling apple brought him the groundbreaking realization that there must be a process like gravity. The structure formula of benzene (he) was found by the German chemist August Kekulé in 1896 in his daily nap. Helmut Kohl and Hans Dietrich Genscher admitted to the reporters that they would not have endured the burdens of politics without a nap in between. Some people stand for a nap, some people conceal it. The British statesman Winston Churchill, known for his clear words, once put it this way:

"Between lunch and dinner you have to sleep, not half things. Take off their clothes and lie down in bed."

Insights from the sleeping laboratories of the world.

Research results clearly show that a nap at noon reduces the risk of myocardial infarction. A short-term sleep during the day can help to increase concentration. But it is not a substitute for night sleep, but rather a refreshment of the mind.

Not only adults benefit from the midday sleep break, it is also beneficial for students. In a study with almost 3,000 schoolchildren in the 4–6th grade in the USA, the results are clear. With a few power naps per week, school performance improved, the children were happier and had fewer behavioral problems.

Catherine E. Milner and Kimberly A. Cot, Brock University, St. Catharines, Ontario, Canada, have looked at the results of many power nap studies and conclude that a short sleep improves mood and improves our well-being and road safety when driving by car.

Marc Rosekind conducted tests on behalf of the US Space Agency NASA to prove that pilots who sleep briefly in between are the better pilots. Their response time is 16% shorter than that of their colleagues. This difference is therefore significant and can make the decisive difference for demanding tasks. The pilots took 5.6 minutes to fall asleep and slept for about 26 minutes. In addition, attention losses decreased by 34%.

A nap increases empathy, as shown in the results of a study by psychologist Ninad Gujar from the University of California in Berkley. The subjects' task was to interpret emotions of faces. The group who had a lunchtime nap evaluated the emotions to choose from, happy, angry and sadly much more positively than those who were without a power nap. The researchers thus prove, among other things, that emotions become more cloudy, the more tired a person is.

Study results of improving the vigilance and performance ability of emergency medical doctors and nurses show that a power nap shows a significant improvement in performance during a 12-hour shift around 03:00 a.m.

Similar results were found in an experiment with aircraft maintenance engineers, who were also allowed to make a recovery sleep of about 20 minutes during the night shift. They were more vigilant afterwards and they were more attentive on the way home.

Lack of sleep makes you less physically and mentally energetic. It could be said that bad sleep leads to a bad mood.

A power nap can counteract it.

Lie down and recharge your confidence!

As shown above, short-term sleep offers many advantages. But it can never replace the night's sleep. During night sleep, the sleep cycles of 90 minutes are passed several times with the four sleep stages. When taking a nap, we usually try not to get into deep sleep at all. And thus, a significant part is missing that is responsible for regeneration, growth and learning.

The graphic explains the differences.

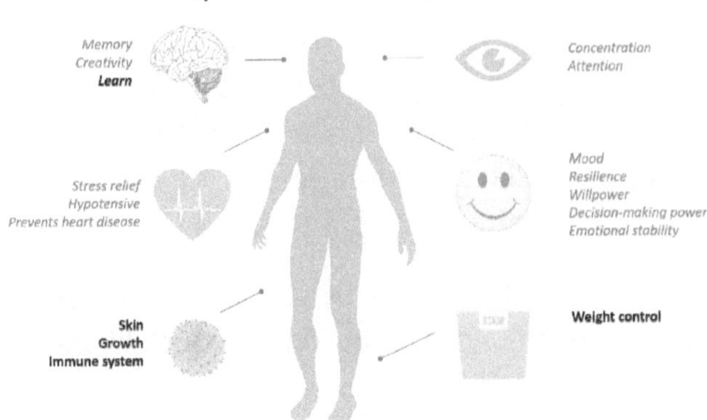

Cultural differences - Inemuri, Siesta and Co.

"Keep 30 minutes free for your worries every day and at this time take a nap."

Abraham Lincoln

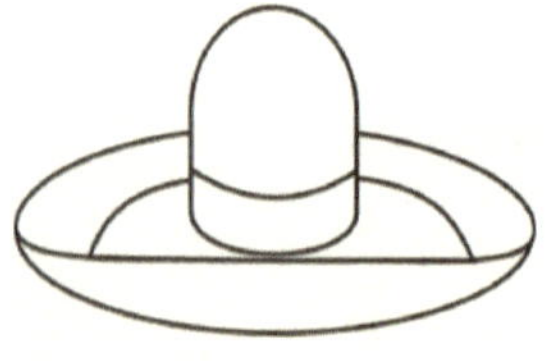 In hot countries, the long lunch break is known as the siesta. Since it is almost impossible to perform normal services in high heat, it is more sustainable to use this time for quiet activities. In South America, three out of four citizens sleep several times a week for up to two hours during the siesta to avoid the heat.

A siesta is not necessarily a power nap, Siesta literally means 6th hour. This generally means lunchtime, which serves as a rest break. A power nap is defined as a short-time sleep of up to 30 minutes.

But it is not dozed all the time. In the word Siesta, many see in spirit the Mexican sit with shadowy sombrero who half obscures man. But reality is different. Driven by globalization, it becomes difficult for many companies to endure such extremely long breaks. Business life is kept alive in air-conditioned rooms. The Spaniards have been trying to soften the rigid siesta from 14:00 –

17:00, since employees can do nothing during this time and therefore come home very late.

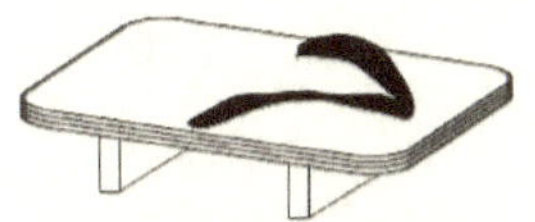 In Asia, there is a true midday sleep culture – a power nap is well known and recognized. In Japan, the doe-sen can be observed in all places and on all (un) possible occasions. People who do not know each other, lean against each other in the subway and sleep. Japan has the shortest sleep time of all industrialized nations: it is less than 6 hours and 20 minutes. From the post-war years to the present day, the bedtime time has shifted from around 22:00 to midnight. Remain is the rising time. So they only get too little sleep and allow themselves an 'inemuri', which means intermediate short-term sleep – i.e. power nap.

In China, sleep is allowed at noon, which is legally protected. In fact, you can meet people in the furniture store who lie down at noon and sleep in front of everyone's eyes (most of them are closed anyway).

The situation is similar in Taiwan. There, the office workers sleep with the doors open. Customers and suppliers are signaled in such a way that it is better to come later.

In the business and industrial centers Taipei, Hong Kong, Singapore, Kuala Lumpur, Saigon, etc., you can hardly feel the standstill in the midday rest, but in the countryside people still live their healthy rhythm and can hardly be stopped from the midday sleep.

Implementation — when, where, how best to do it?

To ensure that the short-term sleep is also restful, one should know the following basic conditions and take them into account. If the power nap hasn't worked so far, check the next pages for explanations and solutions.

When? Is there an optimum power nap time?

Naps should not normally be taken after 15:00 (no shift operation). The reason for this is that the sleep fatigue cannot build up enough until bedtime.

The general recommendation is to place the nap diametral to the middle of sleep. Thus, with a (even sleep-wake rhythm) and a waking time between 06:00 and 09:00 in the morning, the lunchtime between 13:00 and 15:00 is actually the most conducive.

When getting up earlier or later, the slope of wanting to sleep shifts in the same phase, but the REM sleep ability changes less synchronously. The reason for this lies in the already mentioned circadian rhythm (the biological rhythm of the day) and other complex internal processes.

Power Nap works best diametrically to the sleep middle of the night

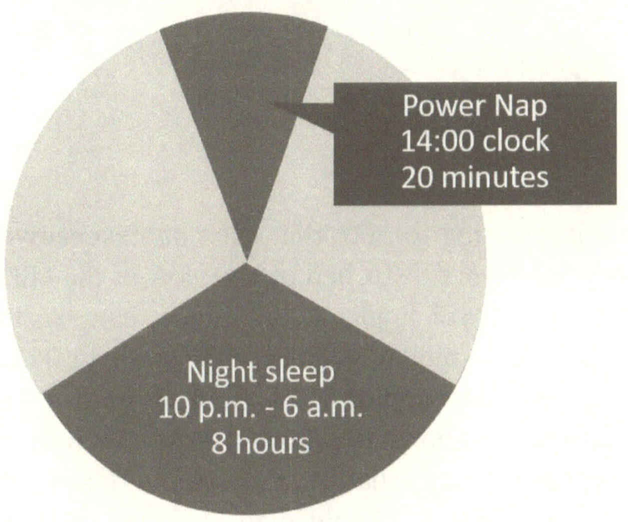

Timing is critical for successful power napping. The American sleep researcher Dr. Sara C. Mednick and her team have explored how exactly this happens. In her 2006 book "Take a Nap", she shows that sleep pressure (fatigue) rises from the moment of getting up over the day until bedtime. This is not surprising, but at the same time the REM sleep ability, which is important for effective short sleep, decreases over the course of the day. And this results in a certain window of time for the optical power nap.

Wake up time

05:30	06:00	06:30	07:00	07:30	08:00	08:30
13:15	13:30	13:45	14:00	14:15	14:30	14:45

Start time Power Nap

It is interesting to note that even light-sensitive people, who are disturbed by the glow of the LED of an electrical appliance at night, can easily manage their midday sleep in bright sunlight. This indicates that napping is planned by nature. In addition, it is known that 80% of mammals have a polyphasic sleep, that is, they nod off several times a day. Why should man be extremely far away from it?

Where? Power napping is possible anywhere

The big advantage of short-term sleep is that you don't need anything wide. Immediate implementation is possible wherever you can sit down and lean. To take a nap on the beach or to doze a few minutes at a mountain hut are well-known phenomena.

At home, it's probably easiest to try a power nap. You know the quiet corners and you can set up your sleeping space comfortably. Darkening, music etc. can be designed according to your own wishes.

At the workplace, the employer can ask whether there are rooms and/or company agreements for short-term sleep. Much has been done since the famous introduction of power nap resting facilities at Vechta City Council in 2000. Companies are increasingly required to provide rooms and special loungers for short-term sleep in offices or on factory premises. Since the recognition of midday sleep is not equally pronounced in the business world, it is worthwhile to take your own initiative. In the course of occupational health management, more and more measures for the maintenance of health and services of employees are being accepted and promoted. What was difficult to imagine as a measure years ago is now ready for implementation. This includes the power nap, which is still an exotic concept for many.

If you wouldn't dare nap in the office, you might also be able to doze in your own car during your break with some pleasant music.

Practice example: because the dancers complained of concentration difficulties, the state ballet Berlin sought solutions. Help came from Professor Ingo Fietze, head of the Sleep Medicine Center of Charité Berlin.

After a three-month measurement of the sleep-wake rhythm, it became apparent that the members of the ensemble do not sleep enough with less than seven hours of sleep per night to survive the training program, rehearsals and performances.

The solution now is that there are soundproofed darkened resting cabins with beds, a massage chair and a feel-good lounger. There, the ensemble members can regenerate themselves between rehearsals or before the performance, for example, with a short sleep.

When travelling, for example by train or plane, the power nap can help you arrive at the destination feeling recovered.

Parking trick: On the go, in car parks or in the company car park you can make yourself comfortable in the car. Listen to relaxing music or do some relaxing exercise. Imagine a timer and enjoy your sleep of success.

Hotels recognized the trend a few years ago, that a nap after a meal can save from the bad form depth. The first were the Americans. They have developed a business model out of the problem and call it day-use-rooms. In many big cities there are various hotel chains that offer this service. You rent a room for 1-2 hours a day, so you can lie down between two appointments, recharge your batteries and still stay in business mode.

There is a Powernap studio in Berlin since 2014. The founder is herself is an enthusiastic power napper and offers power-nap niches at 30 minutes intervals for resting.

Some **airports** provide passengers with relaxation areas where you can sleep. The internet portal sleeping in airports offers an extensive overview of worldwide airports and their offer for relaxation areas and much more. Singapore's Changi Airport is regularly ranked first in the international ranking. There are very pleasant snooze lounges. In Munich and Berlin-Tegel, the German startup napcabs GmbH offers cabins for rent for power napping.

Shiftwork is not easy per se. The body is stressed by the constantly changing recovery and activity times. It is working against the inner clock which can be exhausting. In my book Sleepbook for Shiftworkers I look at the special conditions of shiftworkers and offer tips for a healthy sleep. Night shift workers can take a nap before their night shift to recharge their energy and concentration.

Tips for Business Travelers

We realize that our sleeping habits are deeply rooted in us when we sleep in a foreign environment. People who travel more often can sleep well in unfamiliar beds from the first night. People who almost always stay at home on the other hand often have a more restless sleep on the first night. Researchers attribute this to our state of vigilance. The new environment is initially critically observed. The body releases a little more stress hormones than normal, which makes falling asleep and sleeping throughout the night more difficult. This behavior is a good indication for getting used to a sleep routine.

	Quality of sleep	
Sleeping place	always same bed	frequently changing
At home	good	good
Strange environment	first night restless	good

Book your overnight stay as suitable as possible for your wishes – smokers/non-smokers, quiet location etc. Many people know that rooms close to the stairwell or elevator are usually louder due to running and door sounds. Shoe shine machines and crunched ice machines are also to be avoided because people use these sources of noise at all (un) possible times.

Hotels in a city location should have good soundproofing against traffic noise and still provide sufficient oxygen in the room.

If you arrive during the day, you have enough opportunity to ventilate the room and adjust the temperature to your needs.

- Test the bed to see if it is squeaky, too hard, too soft or too short.

- Does the pillow fit, is it large/small/high/soft enough?

- Is the bed linen warm or cool enough?

- Check if the room can be darkened properly. Semi-transparent curtains can cause some people to wake up very early in summertime.

A walk before going to bed beats the glass of alcohol at the bar. The usual bedtime and the personal de-tension ritual make it easier to fall asleep.

Travel kit checklist:

Earplugs	☐	Medications	☐
Pillow	☐	Ointments/Aromas	☐
Alarm clock	☐	Sleep tea	☐
Music	☐	Notepad + Pen	☐
Eye mask	☐	Skin cream	☐
Socks	☐	Disinfectants	☐
Water bottle	☐	Mosquito repellent	☐
Readings	☐	Towel	☐

How? What is the correct duration?

Until a few years ago, a nap 10-30 minutes in duration was recommended.. The reason for this was that it is often difficult to get yourself up after getting into the deep sleep phase.. The question is whether people wake up by themselves in a deep sleep phase. Isn't it more likely that people who wake up feeling grumpy woke up before or after the deep sleep phase?

It is known today that some people, a few per cent of the population, cannot quite enjoy napping, whether their nap is short or long. The following research results are probably interesting for everyone else.

Are six minutes better than 60 minutes?

Those who want to increase their ability to remember during the day should sleep shorter instead of longer. The subjects who were allowed to sleep for 60 minutes clearly improved their performance compared to those who performed a note test without sleep. Even better, the participants had only six minutes of sleep! An ER-clarification attempt is that the brains of babies and toddlers learn extremely much and, as is known, they insert several short naps a day – the so-called polyphasic sleep. "Only adult people have this monolithic sleep block," explains Dr. Olaf Lahl, scientist at Hein-Rich Heine University Düsseldorf. And he believes that the extremely short sleep time pushes memory retention.

Researchers Amber Brooks and Leon Lack from the School of Flinders University in Australia confirm with their results that 10 minutes of power napping are very effective. They let their subjects sleep for 5, 10, 20, and 30 minutes to find out what the optimal duration is.

The 5-minute nap resulted in few advantages compared to the control without a nap. The 10-

minute nap resulted in an immediate improvement of all endpoints (including sleep delay, subjective drowsiness, fatigue, vitality, and cognitive performance), retaining some of these benefits for 155 minutes. The 20-minute nap was associated with improvements that occurred 35 minutes after the nap and stopped up to 125 minutes after the nap.

Dr. Sarah Mednick and Prof. Dr. Axel Mecklinger, neuropsychologists at the University of Saarland have determined the opposite result in their research. Both researchers highlight the results of 45–60 minute naps.

Mecklinger has proven with his colleagues that a short sleep of about an hour can significantly increase memory performance. The study design was designed to test a real learning of new content. 41 volunteers learned nonsensical words and pairs of words. Subsequently, the learning content was checked. After that, half of the participants were allowed to take a power nap. Meanwhile, the others watched a DVD. The sleepers were clearly ahead of the second test, they remembered much better.

"A short sleep of 45 to 60 minutes improves memory by a factor of five,"

explains Axel Mecklinger.

Sarah Mednick believes that the better results of the longer naps could be due to the fact that REM sleep phases may be included. On the other hand, the brain gets into slower vibrations during deeper sleep phases. The lower working frequency (slow-wave-sleep, SWS) is also associated with memory consolidation (learning and remembering).

One conclusion that can be drawn from the research is that napping in the workplace, university or school significantly improves learning success.

These findings also suggest that people should find out what sleeping practices work for themselves. For example, some people are able to nap for only 15 minutes and wake up feeling refreshed, whereas others require the use of an alarm clock to wake them up.

The graph shows a sleep cycle as it occurs in natural night sleep. A sleep cycle with all four sleep phases takes about 90 minutes. From falling asleep to reaching deep sleep, about 30 minutes pass. The first phase of deep sleep lasts the longest and becomes shorter from time to time. The duration of REM sleep on the other hand tends to increase with each cycle.

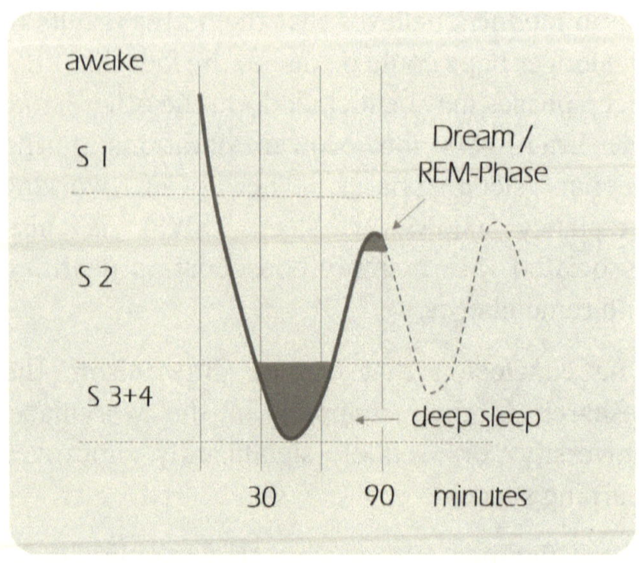

Research also shows that a 30 minute deep sleep as well as REM sleep parts can be seen in power naps. Sleep has an idiosyncratic structure.

Chapter 2 Prepare your naps well and effectively

General:

If you do not know your optimal short-term sleep duration, read the tips in Chapter 3.

Prepare your environment:

It does not hurt to give your Power Nap the best chance for success. The prerequisite for this is to worry about the implementation. Therefore, try to eliminate all sorts of disturbing factors so that you can fall asleep and rest.

1. Light

One tip for falling asleep to work faster is to provide a sense of darkness, as naps are usually taken during the day. Darkness helps particularly sensitive people to fall asleep faster. This is certainly easier at home than in the office. A sleep mask is best suited here. This can also be taken inconspicuously anywhere, as it fits in any pocket.

2. Noise

There are different types of people: some can only fall asleep when it is completely silent. Even the smallest noise is disturbing here. Others on the other hand may be able to nod off in a crowded subway train. Everyone has to find the best way to switch off briefly in a suitable relocation.

In the office, it may be too loud and you just can't relax. In cases like these, it may help to listen to relaxing music with headphones. Many also find a monotonous sound such as white noise or rain pleasant enough to fall asleep to.

3. Air

Odors, but also the air or room temperature are also factors which affect the likelihood of falling asleep.

Room temperature is also a factor when it comes to falling asleep in general. If it's too cold or too hot, you can't help but focus on it which prevents you from falling asleep.

4. Location

A power nap is a form of short-term sleep as described previously. Therefore, it is recommended to perform it while sitting. It should still be comfortable and sleepy. In the office, it is ideal if you sit down and put your head on your crossed arms at your desk. If there is an extra room in the office where you can relax, then of course it should be preferred. Some of these rooms have armchairs in which you can safely sit back and be completely to yourself. Regardless of the situation, it is still crucial that the starting position is comfortable.

Lying, the natural sleeping position, is of course just as well suited. But most people need a location in which they feel comfortable. A lockable room is optimal here.

Setting an alarm is always an advantage, as it reminds you that the maximum 30 minutes have expired and you should definitely get up because the rhythm plays a big role here.

Tips for falling asleep

For people who naturally need a long time to fall asleep, the following exercises can help you to fall asleep faster. The following exercises have been proven time and time again to promote relaxation. In addition, these exercises can also be performed at intervals during the day, helping to lower your stress level. Proven methods are autogenic training, imaginary journey, progressive muscle relaxation, yoga and self-hypnosis.

By performing these exercises regularly, you will notice that it is always easier for you to fall into a short sleep. It is recommended to set an alarm clock to 30 minutes so that you do not oversleep and at the same time get used to the rhythm.

1. Muscle relaxation + suggestion

Focus on one part of the body, for example, your right hand. Inhale, then tighten your fist vigorously for five seconds. Then let go and exhale. After about 30 seconds, switch to the next part of the body, for example, to the left hand. Inhale, then tighten your fist vigorously for five seconds. Then let go and exhale. After about 30 seconds, switch to the next part of the body. Continue until all parts of the body have been strained. Last but not least, you tighten the whole body. This exercise works just as well as in the lying gene.

The following exercise is an example from autogenic training.

Concentrate on your left arm and say, "My arm is getting heavy, very heavy, ever heavier." Repeat this until you feel that your arm has become heavy. Then focus on your right arm and repeat.

Now, when the right arm is sleeping, continue with your feet in the same way. After that, the legs become heavy. The torso is getting heavy. Everything feels heavy, the whole body is heavy and tired and is looking forward to sleep.

2. Breathe

By focusing on your breathing, the stressful everyday life and disturbing thoughts can be briefly hidden.

Breathing is probably the oldest, easiest and at the same time safest way to relax. The colloquial well-known tip, simply taking a deep breath or taking a deep breath in case of trouble, brings it almost to the point. For breathing to have a relaxing effect, it is important to exhale longer than usual. Most men usually breathe far too flatly. This is especially noticeable in stressful situations. It is inhaled and exhaled only in the upper chest area.

The special trick that leads to calming is the long exhalation up to max. 3-4 seconds.

In this exercise, it is important to inhale for 3-4 seconds, briefly hold the air and exhale slowly. One only draws attention to it and becomes calmer. It might be possible that you don't even know how to fall asleep at the beginning, but if you power nap regularly, you get a feeling for it.

Even if initially it should not work out with sleep, after a maximum of 30 minutes, get up and move. The body is learning this rhythm and can get used to it. Even without sleep, the short break brings a knowledgeable success. You could relax and focused only on yourself during this time. Thus, one approaches oneself again and pays more attention to the physical signals. With some exercise, it will always be easier to make a short-term sleep and be relaxed. If you control the power nap, you don't even need an alarm clock in the long run. The inner clock will then signal when it's time to get up to work, which you will be able to do more efficiently and in a more relaxed state of mind.

3. Fantasy rods

There are no limits to the power napper here. Whether you think of a day in the land of milk and honey, bathe in money or win a prize as a star architect – everything is possible. The following scene on the beach is an example of a calming story. It works well when you get involved in it – so you can introduce yourself to the beach with all your senses.

"Imagine you're on the beach. You're enjoying watching the movement of the waves as they crash on the seashore. You listen to the rhythmic sounds going on around you. You feel the wind brush your skin. The fresh scent of the sea soothes. The warm fine-grained sand invites you to sit down. It's nice to be there watching the surf. The sea comes and goes in its eternal, uniform and soothing rhythm. Whenever any distracting thoughts appear, you gently return to the seaside scene."

You can also use other relaxation exercises. Do what works for you. Special music such crashing waves or rain falling helps many people to switch off. The quiet trickling in the background does not distract too much, but gives a comfortable, soothing or at least neutral feeling.

Every stressful situation has a history! Therefore, check which stress can be avoided by preventive care.

Often unfortunate circumstances coincide with each other. With hindsight, we note that some things could have been avoided if we had approached the matter with more calm. In case of recurring activities, advance planning and organization may help you to avoid unnecessary stress. Sometimes simple thinking or asking someone for advice is enough to eliminate possible sources of stress from the outset.

Ask yourself:

WHERE can I start today to avoid stress?

Another good way to reduce stress is to focus on something other than stress. This may not work immediately in every situation, but it does work eventually.

Ask yourself:

Who can I bring joy to today?

These two questions have helped many thousands of people to experience the day differently, in other words better. And every person who carries a bit more ingenious serenity has a relaxing and beneficial effect on his environment.

Barbara Fredrickson, researcher in the field of positive psychology, describes in her book "positivity" a simple experiment with high impact. Test subjects who watched a funny film for one minute processed stressful situations emotionally as well as physically fast. Among other things, heart rate variability was measured, which shows a fast and yet accurate determination of the physiology. So sometimes it doesn't take much to get into a good mood.

How to wake up without an alarm clock

These tricks help you to wake up even without an alarm clock.

Key trick:

Einstein's recipe: He probably knew about the refreshing effect of a creative nap. He sat down and placed a keychain in his hand. At the moment deep relaxation, his muscles loosened and he woke up from the sound of the falling keys. If there is carpet in the office, you can place a plate in the place where the key will fall when you release it. The sound makes you wake up pretty fast.

Truck driver trick:

Truck drivers lean on the steering wheel with their upper body and let their arms hang loosely. When dozing away, a stagnation of blood is formed in the hands, they begin to tingle heavily. It's not for everyone, but it works.

Caffeine Kick Trick

You should never drink coffee before going to bed, but here it is strongly recommended. The stimulating effect of coffee actually happens only after 20 minutes. Therefore, it is perfect to drink some before taking a power nap. The caffeine then boosts circulation at the appropriate time. Because you are not only rested after the short-term sleep, but also fresh and cheerful.

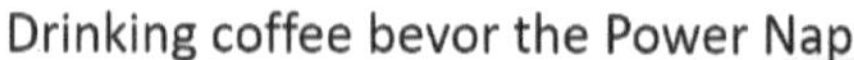

Drinking coffee bevor the Power Nap

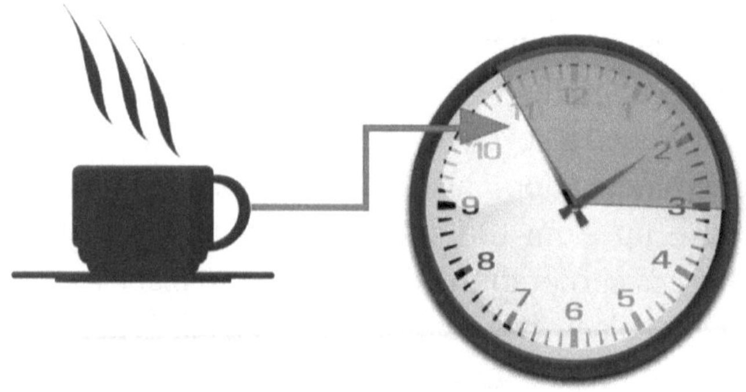

Neck Trick:

You can also sleep while sitting with your head not leaning. After about 15 to 20 minutes, the muscles of the neck relax, the head falls to the side and you wake up.

Activation after a power nap

Become active immediately after the power nap. That's an important rule. Anyone who stays lying down and simply continues to doze may give away the recovery effect. Instead of indulging in leisure, it is part of the Power Nap to get going immediately afterwards.

Man reacts to environmental stimuli and this can be exploited when waking up after a nap. Interessant for our biosystem is light: we automatically look where it is brighter. This has long been known in sales psychology. Stores illuminate certain zones or goods to be brighter in order to deliberately control where customers walk. Change your sleeping place to the light – preferably to the sunlight. This and the following tricks will help you get ready not only after nap at noon, but also in the morning faster.

Movement is the best activator. After your power nap, start with simple, light arm and leg movements. Have a good stretch, but not too violently, to prevent dizziness. Increase in-game activity by bouncing or a virtual boxing match. After 2-3 minutes, the circulation is in motion and the brain is fully ready for use.

Climbing stairs or walking around the block helps to gradually wake you up again. This will also help you get some fresh air and sunlight.

Nutrition is a key stimulus. A glass of water with lemon slices, mint and ginger invigorates and refreshes. Eating an apple or chewing a gum will also help to wake you up.

Social contacts can only be maintained in the waking state. After a short-term sleep, approach other people.

Getting through simple tasks and working creatively is especially easy for many people after a nap.

Top tip:

Although washing your face helps you to feel refreshed, it can also energize you. What our grandparents always told us, Stress researchers confirmed in their studies.

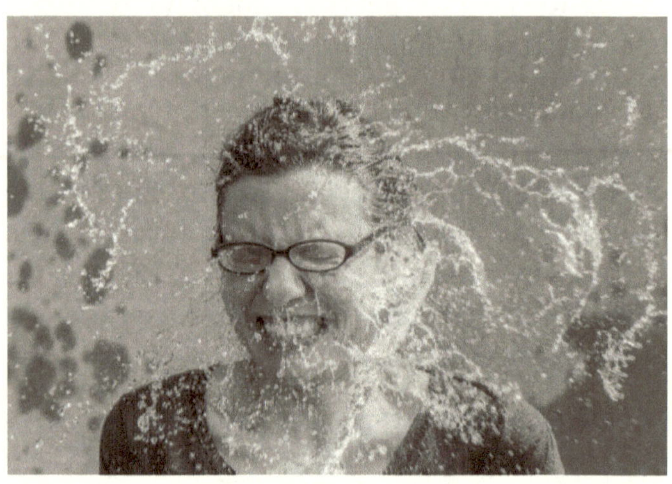

Chapter 3 Power Napping: Tips and Tricks

If you do not know exactly how long your optimal power nap duration is, then start this experiment under the best possible conditions. You should look for a dark and quiet place where you won't be disturbed.

Power Nap: Everything speaks for it — no mind, so you should take care of your daily lunch sleep.

How to find your optimal power nap duration

Schedule your power nap between 13:00 and 15:00 and set an alarm clock for 30 minutes.

Lie down and try not to think about anything special. Be mindful of your breath and then just doze away.

Wake up before the alarm signal, then activate immediately. Get up and get a drink, for example, a glass of water. If you are fit and cheerful after a few minutes, then this is your natural duration for a power nap.

If you are awakened by the alarm clock, you also activate as describe how you feel.

If your perceived fitness level is less than 5 on a subjective scale of 1 (tired) to 10 (high energy) then reduce your sleep time in five-minute steps with power naps in the next few days. In this experiment, do only one power nap per day.

Write down the results in the following table.

Date	Time	Duration	Fitness	Other

Result:

My optimal short-term sleep duration is...
Minutes:

My optimal Power Nap time is around:

_______a.m /_______p.m

Skillfully Power Nap — these are the rules!

The three main success factors for short-term sleep:

- Start your personal Power Nap before 15:00 so that you can fall asleep well at night.

- Be sure to set an alarm clock so that you do not sleep for more than 30 minutes.

- Get up immediately after napping and become active.

Find a quiet spot and take a refreshing nap daily.

First aid for sleepiness when driving

Fatigue when driving is a big issue when you have to travel long distances. Driving when tired is dangerous because accidents occur again and again due to the so-called second sleep. It is essential to avoid falling asleep at the wheel. Just 1.5 seconds of micro-sleep at a speed of 120 km/h mean having travelled 50 meters blind. 50 meters is a huge distance if you drift out of lane or the vehicle in front suddenly breaks. Even if you awake immediately, you still need a reaction time to assess the situation correctly and act adequately. 17 hours without sleep has the effect of 0.05% alcohol in the blood. Thus, being awake for too long significantly reduces response time.

Pay attention to these typical body signals which are a sign of overfatigue:

- The eyes begin to burn and become heavy.

- The environment becomes blurred. You experience double vision.

- Keeping track is difficult.

- You start daydreaming.

- You miss traffic signs etc.

- Your response time slows down.

- You yawn and you change sitting position more often.

Fatigue at the wheel must not be underestimated: what often goes well can have sudden catastrophic consequences. That's why it's always a good idea to have a passenger who can keep their eye on the driver, or even better, alternate. Oftentimes time pressure influences decisions on when to drive, but you should always keep this question in mind: is it worth the risk?

Making sure you have enough to eat and drink and giving yourself small breaks and time to exercise can prolong your attention span. Power naps are ideal for longer trips.

Plan a break from the outset for journeys over long distances. Treat yourself to several stops when driving at night. In this case, many stops actually helps a lot.

The Sleep Research Laboratory, Loughborough, University, Leicestershire, England, has conducted experiments with caffeine, placebo and power napping. Compared to just taking a break and power napping, the subjects were attentive much longer after a short sleep and felt less fatigue. Even better results were achieved by the people who first took caffeine and then power napped.

**Be honest with yourself
and behave responsibly.**

Daily energy management: use circadian rhythms

Since the recent scientific breakthrough on circadian rhythms by Nobel Prize-winning chronobiologists, it is clear that there is a deeper meaning to our bodies' own ticking clocks.Nature, for example, has arranged it in such a way that we humans are more sensitive to pain in the morning than after lunch break. This knowledge can be used, for example, to schedule dental appointments at lunchtime.Moreover, this particular time of day is considered best for dentists as coordination and reaction times are optimal.

In terms of power napping, it can be useful to determine your own personal chronotype (early bird vs. night owl) when figuring out the best time to sleep. For those who prefer to stay up late, a power nap after 15.00 is usually fine as they go to bed later and can build up enough sleep pressure until then.

An interesting observation is that sports events are usually set up in the afternoon. This clearly depends on the personal daily form, the possible performance, the regeneration phases, but also on the inner clock of the athletes. In the following graphic you can clearly see that peak human fitness occurs at around 16:00.

The following graphic explains the internal processes.

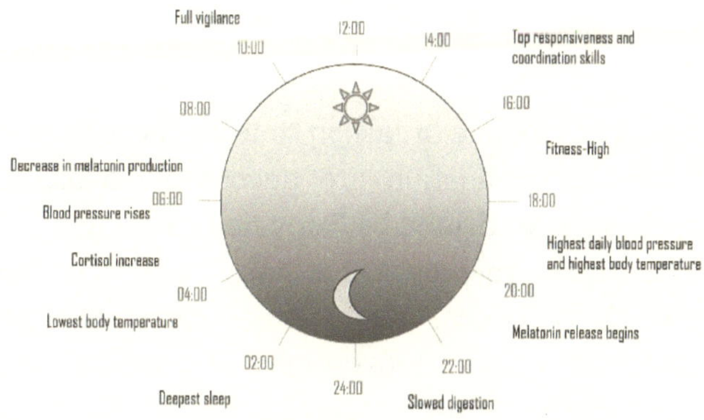

Our daily internal processes follow a biological patternabout 90 minutes duration. This pattern is very similar to the Basic Rest Activity Cycle (BRAC) approach, as it occurs during night sleep. Professor Nathaniel Kleitmann discovered that the body undergoes phases of increased and decreased concentracy capacity.

"Man is a rhythmic being," says occupational scientist Dr. Martin Braun. Therefore, it is necessary to create a balance between the working world and relaxation. The best ideas rarely come at your desk. Only when you relax, leave the workplace and ignore upcoming tasks for a short time can you continue with full energy again. Therefore, minor breaks should be the rule.

The psychology professor at Florida State University K. Anders Ericsson has revealed in his research on memory enhancement that high performers require 90 minutes and then take a break.

The trick is to take breaks in time, because longer periods of exhaustion are necessarily avoided. This is also confirmed by Tony Schwartz, head of https://theenergyproject.com. In an article in the New York Times, he writes that since he embarked on four to five hours of concentrated work a day (with interim breaks after 90 minutes), he has achieved more than before in 10-12 hours of work.

These collected insights help to better structure the working day by adhering to the natural rhythms of the body. People who did not find enough rest during the night and during the day also found that their performance (psychologically, mentally and physically) quickly went downhill.

Relaxation Planner Trick

Whether it's an Outlook or paper calendar, a regular power nap is best done when it's in the appointment calendar. I tell my clients to schedule their power naps three weeks in advance, because they are more easily seen. Since the appointment calendar is a high priority among most people this method works quite well. Even if only three out of five power naps are performed a week, this is a good approach and helps to integrate the mini-sleep breaks into the week.

In addition to planning the nap, I also recommend the inclusion of several short breaks throughout the day. Every mini break gives the body a chance to regenerate and helps to slow down the flow of thoughts.

Tip for implementation: You do not necessarily have to add your napping time to your company calendar which may be seen by hundreds of colleagues. It may be more appropriate to disguise it with something more cryptic, such as an abbreviation, etc.

If you regularly perform relaxation training sessions, even if theylast only five minutes, your stress levels may decrease noticeably after a short period of time. This can also help improve your naps. This is a win-win – your day will be overall more relaxed and your power nap will be more restful.

Known problems and solutions (FAQ)

I do not feel rested. I wake up still feeling exhausted.

If you've tried Power Napping before, you know that after waking up you can feel groggy and more tired than before.

Remedy usually manages to shorten the duration. If you need two hours you should try it with 90 minutes. This is the natural length of a sleep cycle with all four sleep phases. Ideally, you wake up in the so-called REM phase (Rapid Eye Movement) and are ready to go immediately.

Anyone who sleeps about an hour should try out what personal fitness looks like after 30 minutes of sleep. Chapter 4 describes the determination of the optimal individual power nap duration.

I am a shiftworker and take my nap in the evening before starting my night shift. Is that okay?

Yes, this is a good way to counteract sleepiness in the middle of the night, especially between 02:00 and 04:00. Even if you have 2-3 sleep cycles in the morning after your night shift, the Power Nap is a good addition in afternoon.

I usually need 20 minutes to fall asleep - should Shall I add these minutes to my Power Nap duration?

Yes and no. If you have enough time, set your alarm clock to 30 minutes from the moment you lay down. If you wake up to the alarm, that's your time span.

However, if you have only a 20 minute lunch break, it is recommended to do some relaxation exercises as a sleeping aid, as it can be difficult to fall asleep on command.

If you are not familiar with yoga, autogenic training or other relaxation exercises, then you may find it difficult to do at the beginning. Therefore, at the beginning one should start with an easy to learn exercise. The so-called PMR (Progressive Muscle Relaxation) is suitable for this purpose. This is also used to ease stress, sleep disturbances, muscle tension or pain. PMR has a full-body effect and is not only used for relaxation purposes. When you are just starting to explore PMR, it is important to look for a quiet place and concentrate on yourself in order to gain a better sense of your own body. For methodological examples, see Chapter 3.

I can't fall asleep because my job is so hectic.

Falling asleep at the touch of a button can be difficult. In order to put a stop to racing thoughts as you lie in bed at night, you should get used to scheduling defined rest breaks in your daily routine. 2-3 minutes of relaxation performed several times a day can noticeably reduce stress levels.

I could sleep all day – a power nap is not enough for me.

A feeling of fatigue during the day can have different causes. A few days of poor quality or a lack of sleep can cause increased drowsiness during the day. If fatigue persists for a significantly long period of time, the following causes may be considered:

• sleep deficit, overexertion on your body, vitamin and/or mineral deficiency, disease, hormonal shifts, winter blues, mental state

If you are experiencing 2-3 weeks of insomnia it is advisable to consult a doctor to clarify the causes. In the case of more severe sleep disturbances, participating in a sleep study may be a good measure to overcome sleeping difficulties and obtain a diagnosis.

Author

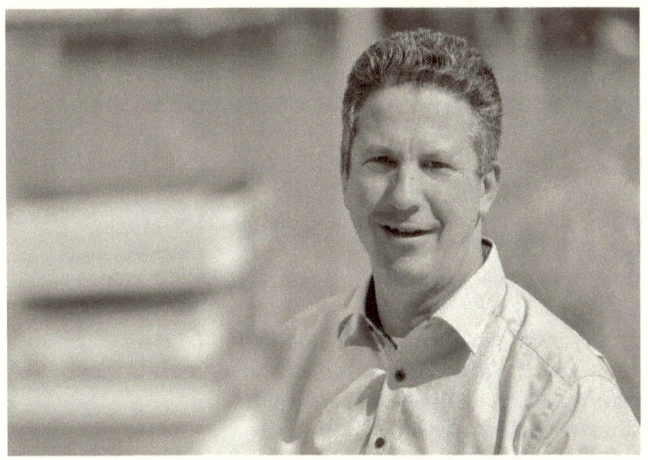

Author, consultant, coach and trainer.

Klaus Kampmann, born in 1962 near Stuttgart, has gained over 20 years of experience as a technical officer of international marketing and training in a technology company.

Since 2006 he has been the owner of Kampmann Coaching and, as an expert for positive personal development and sleep, supports people in all levels in organizations.

His work conveys working concepts that can be learned within a short time and have a lasting effect. He is known for his appearances in TV, radio and newspapers. Numerous customer references (e.g. DAX-100 and DOW-30 companies) confirm the high effectiveness of Kampmann's methods.

Research

https://www.ncbi.nlm.nih.gov/pubmed/17765011
https://www.researchgate.net/publication/15581165_Postprandial_
Sleep_in_Healthy_Men
https://academic.oup.com/sleep/advance-article-
abstract/doi/10.1093/sleep/zsz126/5499200?redirectedFrom=fullte
xt
https://onlinelibrary.wiley.com/doi/epdf/10.1111/j.1365-
2869.2008.00718.x
https://onlinelibrary.wiley.com/doi/pdf/10.1111/j.1365-
2869.1995.tb00229.x
https://www.sciencedaily.com/releases/2009/06/090610091343.ht
m
https://www.ncbi.nlm.nih.gov/pubmed/17052562
https://www.hotel.de/blog/mittagsschlaf-in-deutschen-hotels/
https://www.nickerchen-berlin.de/power-of-nap
https://www.sleepinginairports.net/
https://www.napcabs.com/
https://www.uni-duesseldorf.de/home/infocenter-
hhu/aktuell/archivmeldungen/archivmeldungen-
detailansicht/article/schon-ein-kurzer-schlaf-hat-positive-
auswirkungen.html
https://www.ncbi.nlm.nih.gov/pubmed/16796222
https://www.uni-
saarland.de/nc/en/university/news/article/nr/12337.html
https://www.uni-
saarland.de/nc/en/university/news/article/nr/12337.html
https://www.ncbi.nlm.nih.gov/pubmed/12819785
Fredrickson, Barbara: die macht der guten gefühle, Campus, 2011,
S.133
https://www.sciencedirect.com/science/article/pii/S1388245703002
554
https://www.ncbi.nlm.nih.gov/pubmed/8936399
https://www.btq.de/fileadmin/btq/media/Artikel/cua6_09_20_24.p
df
https://www.nytimes.com/2013/02/10/opinion/sunday/relax-youll-
be-more-productive.html?_r=1

www.ingramcontent.com/pod-product-compliance
Lightning Source LLC
Chambersburg PA
CBHW051236250726
48655CB00006B/2803